YOU CAN SPEAK AGAIN

*A Guide to Speech after
a Laryngectomy*

YOU CAN
SPEAK AGAIN

A Guide to Speech after a Laryngectomy

By Charles R. Nelson

Revised and Updated
by Joan Steen Wilentz

Funk & Wagnalls
NEW YORK

Manufactured in the United States of America

1 2 3 4 5 6 7 8 9 10

Library of Congress Cataloging in Publication Data

Nelson, Charles R
    You can speak again.

        First ed. published in 1949 under title:
        Post-laryngectomy speech.
        I. Esophageal speech I. Wilentz, Joan Steen.
II. Title.
RF540.N44   1976   617'.533   76-16513
ISBN 0-308-10257-6
ISBN 0-308-10260-6 (pbk.)

Contents

Contents

Preface to the Second Edition

CHARLES NELSON WAS a pioneer in the methods of teaching post-laryngectomy speech. In his generation, few were taught in a formal way. The general advice was "Start talking—just go ahead and do it!" Nelson did, and then went on to analyze what he was doing so that he could teach others. Like many gifted teachers he was ever encouraging and optimistic, sympathetic to the problems of the post-operative patient as only one who has experienced surgery himself can be.

He knew that progress in relearning speech was not a matter of "every day in every way getting better and better." There were times when the voice was strong and clear,

times when it was less so. But he knew that with patience
and practice the student could become a good esophageal
speaker. During the course of his career he was associated
with the Alfred Dixon Speech Systems, Inc., in New York
City, the New York University-Bellevue Medical Center
(now simply New York University Medical Center) and the
New York Eye and Ear Infirmary.

The first edition of this book appeared in 1949, making it
one of the earliest manuals of instruction available to the
laryngectomized person. Since then, speech pathologists
and others conducting research in speech and hearing have
analyzed the speech patterns and photographed the positions and movements of the tongue, lips, throat, and
esophagus of laryngectomized speakers. As a result they
have been able to distinguish among inhalation and the
various glossal press or injection methods of air intake.
Rather than champion one method over another, speech
therapists generally favor an eclectic point of view: Let the
student try a variety of methods and see which is most
comfortable for him or her. That is why a chapter entitled
"Esophageal Speech—The Ways and Means" has been
added to the Second Edition. It is followed by a description
of the method Nelson himself employed and taught. But as
he said then, and we repeat now, the important thing to do
is to get air in and control it for speech. If one method works
better for you, by all means use it and don't worry about any
of the others.

Changes and additions to the text have also been made in
the chapter on personal health care—"Some Dos and
Don'ts"; in the chapter on artificial larynges; and in the
discussion of the feelings of the patient and the reactions of

others—"Insight and Outlook." This again is because more research has been done and more practical advice and equipment are available (stoma bibs, shower guards, and so on). The number of personal anecdotes has been increased to include more recent case histories.

For the rest, the lesson plans and readings are much as Nelson laid them out. The gradual buildup of vocal ability from vowels or simple consonant-vowel syllables to longer and more difficult language elements is sound pedagogy. So is the advice to relax, not to overdo to the point of strain, and to curb those faults common to beginners early, before they become entrenched as habits. Those principles and admonitions were essential to the learning process then and continue to be standard procedure in speech-training centers today.

JOAN STEEN WILENTZ

Acknowledgments

I WISH TO THANK Drs. John P. Ruppe and Maxwell D. Ryan of the New York Eye and Ear Infirmary, and the Hon. Eugene G. Schulz, Justice, Court of Special Sessions in New York City. But for them this book might never have been written.

For their kindness in giving me the opportunity of employing my method of learning to speak again, I extend my gratitude to Drs. Howard A. Rusk, George G. Deaver, John F. Daly, and Samuel S. Sverdlik of New York University-Bellevue Medical Center, and Mr. Alfred Dixon of Alfred Dixon Speech Systems.

To the following persons, for their reading of the text of

this book in the manuscript stage and for helpful suggestions, I acknowledge my indebtedness: Drs. Einar Sunde, Hans Christensen, and Howard Bancks of the Methodist Hospital, Brooklyn, N. Y.; Drs. Nathan Blanckfield and Edward Shapiro of Brooklyn, N. Y.; Dr. Franklyn B. Theis of Nyack Hospital; Dr. Jane Dorsey Zimmerman of Columbia University; the E.N.T. surgeons of the New York Eye and Ear Infirmary, Kings County Hospital, and New York University-Bellevue Medical Center; Mr. James J. O'Connell of the Department of English, Bayside High School, Bayside, N. Y.; and Miss Ann Nelson, my sister, of the New Jersey College for Women, New Brunswick, New Jersey.

I also acknowledge with appreciation the cooperation given me by the library staffs of the Metropolitan Life Insurance Company and the New York Academy of Medicine. My best thanks are expressed to Sgt. Thomas E. Creighton and the officers and men of the 1st Q. M. Truck Co., N. Y. G., for giving me, when I needed it most, their unselfish and understanding comradeship. To the unknown taxicab driver whose insulting remarks instilled in me the determination to speak again, I offer my heartfelt thanks. And to my wife, Lillian, I acknowledge with deep gratitude her continuous smile and cheerfulness. Finally, I wish to thank my pupils who, by their acceptance of my method of learning to speak again and by their efforts to rehabilitate themselves, gave me the courage and the desire to prepare this book.

CHARLES R. NELSON

Acknowledgments for the Second Edition

I WANT TO EXPRESS my gratitude to the many students in speech classes for laryngectomees that I observed or attended. Their perseverance, graciousness, and good humor were impressive and inspiring. Some were new students in private sessions with a speech therapist. Others were in intermediate groups, improving breath control and articulation. One advanced class was working on speech rhythms and inflection, learning the effective use of pauses and of rising and falling intonation for greater emphasis and clarity of expression.

The youngest student I saw was a state trooper in his thirties, who was just beginning speech lessons. He was delighted to find that a standard police whistle could be fitted with a ring to fit over the stoma to produce a fine strong whistle. The oldest was a man in his eighties, who had decided to come back for a refresher course. In addition to native Americans, there were Chinese- and Spanish-speaking students, a number of European-born, and some West Indians, who spoke with the lilting cadences of Caribbean English.

Some were teachers, some lawyers, one pursuing a career in politics. Another was a well-known dramatic coach. There were housewives, dietitians, secretaries, businessmen, writers, manual laborers.

Some had begun to say their first words within days of surgery. Others reported that it took them weeks or even months before the first sounds emerged. The most extraordinary case history was that of a World War II veteran whose laryngectomy came about as a result of wounds and infection. He had spent twenty-six years in a convalescent home and had never learned how to speak. When it was discovered that there was no physical deterrent, he was enrolled in a course at a local university and within a short time he, too, had relearned speech—possibly a record for years of silence.

I want also to thank the speech teachers for letting me interview them and watch them in action. Some were professional speech pathologists and therapists. Others were laryngectomized persons—excellent speakers who had had additional training to become instructors. Their demonstrable talent was a powerful incentive and reinforcing agent toward learning at all levels of achievement.

I particularly want to thank the staff of the Speech and

Hearing Institute of the ICD Rehabilitation and Research Center in New York City: the speech pathologists Elaine Harris and Rosalie Braunstein, and the four laryngectomized instructors, John McClear, Clara Koenig, Frank Favorini, and Salvatore Aloisi. John McClear, a distinguished and gifted teacher, is himself an author of a text on post-laryngectomy speech, and an example of the rare individual who has had to relearn speech twice—the second occasion as a result of complications leading to a second bout of surgery.

In addition to those teachers and other therapists I interviewed in New York City, I want to thank Robert F. Nagel, Assistant Clinical Professor of Otolaryngology, Yale University School of Medicine, New Haven, Connecticut, and Dan Kelly, Associate Professor of Communication Disorders and Coordinator of the Voice Clinic at Southern Connecticut State College, also in New Haven.

I must also thank Doctor John F. Daly, Chairman of the Department of Otolaryngology, New York University School of Medicine, who reviewed the medical and surgical aspects of laryngectomy for me, and also in New York City, Jack L. Ranney, Executive Secretary of the International Association of Laryngectomees and members of the staff of the American Cancer Society. They provided me with background material, screened films, and otherwise acquainted me with the services and educational programs of the two societies.

In addition to observing esophageal speech classes, I was fortunate to see demonstrations of and experiment with artificial larynges. These gave me some idea of the problems of phrasing and articulation the laryngectomized person faces. I tried to master esophageal voice myself, inspired by students and also by a number of normal-voiced instructors who can demonstrate esophageal voice using a variety of techniques. It's not easy to do when you have normal vocal cords, and I have not yet succeeded. All the more reason, then, why I must humbly concur with the amused laryngectomee student I saw in an advanced speech class. At the end of the session he turned to me and said with a smile and a mildly self-satisfied air: "We can talk like you—but you can't talk like us!"

JOAN STEEN WILENTZ

YOU CAN SPEAK AGAIN

A Guide to Speech after a Laryngectomy

Laryngectomy

THE PURPOSE of this book is to serve the needs of the thousands of men and women who have been forced each year to give up their natural voice. This is because a disorder, usually cancer, has necessitated surgery for the removal of the larynx, or voice box as it is sometimes called.

You have been blessed with two legs, two arms, and two ears. If something should go wrong with any one of these parts, you would still have the second one to fall back upon. Your larynx, too, contains a pair of parts: two vocal cords. Sometimes surgery spares one of the cords, and in that case you can speak almost normally, relying on the remaining cord. But in most cases both vocal cords are removed. When that happens, you must use other parts of your body and your remaining speaking apparatus as a substitute for your old voice.

To do this, you have to learn a new way of talking. It is to help you master this skill that this book has been written. Anyone who is not severely handicapped, who really wants to speak again, and who follows the principles and methods explained in the text should be able to. The only person who may not is the person who won't try.

We will not discuss medical matters in the text to any great extent. We feel that this should be left to the professionals. Too much harm has been done by people who try to prescribe for others when they themselves lack the necessary training. What the author does know, because of his own experience in having a laryngectomy, is that anyone who undergoes this operation can return to a normal life in a short time if he or she is willing to.

The author also knows, from the actual experience of restoring speech to himself and to many others, that you, too, can regain speech. The human body is a sounding board. By showing you how to use that sounding board to best advantage, you can obtain a voice that is pleasant and distinct. As a result of my own personal experience in learning speech and in teaching others, I know the problems that confront you. I can pass on to you the understanding, assurance, and knowledge that you most need at this time.

Your voice is not a piece of mechanical equipment that can be left at a repair shop with instructions for it to be mended. It is a part of you. The effort you put into it to make it perfect is entirely up to you.

The lifesaving operation the surgeon performed on you was unknown a generation or two ago, and many people were left uncured. Today, with modern surgical techniques, sometimes accompanied by radiation therapy, the operation of laryngectomy is a proven success. Thousands of people owe their good health and long lives to the surgeons who have made this possible through their tireless labors and research.

How did it happen?

Most likely, you were troubled by hoarseness, on and off, for a long time. There were occasions when you couldn't speak above a whisper. You may or may not have had any pain, not even a sore throat. You may have cut down on smoking or given it up entirely and were doctoring yourself for what you thought was a case of laryngitis. But somehow the hoarseness persisted, and your voice didn't sound right.

Finally you got up the courage to see a doctor—most likely a general practitioner. He looked at your throat and suggested you see a throat specialist. The specialist gave your throat a thorough examination. He used mirrored instruments, felt all around the neck area, and took X rays. He told you that there appeared to be a small growth on your larynx. He recommended a minor operation (a biopsy) to allow him to remove a piece of the growth for microscopic examination.

A few days later you returned to his office and were told that the analysis showed that the growth was cancerous and an operation for the removal of the larynx was necessary. He explained that this removal would leave you without voice, but that in time you could learn to speak again without a larynx. He also told you that a small opening would be left in your neck, called a stoma (which means hole), through which you would breathe.

Naturally this news came as a great shock to you, and you felt that it was the end of everything. If you survived the operation at all, you would be disfigured. You'd have a hole in your neck for everyone to see, and what's more, you would be mute. None of this was true. The operation itself is one of the safest procedures surgeons perform. What you were imagining was far worse than the reality. After the laryngectomy you would discover that the stoma could be neatly covered, leaving you free to breathe in comfort; no one would notice it. You also would realize that recovery from the surgery is routine and you would feel well enough to be up and around in short order. Finally you would come to understand that you could learn to speak again. In short, if you heeded your doctor's advice and went ahead with the surgery, you would be on the road to a ripe old age. If you didn't, only tragedy could result.

You agreed to undergo the operation, and the arrangements were made for your hospitalization. Precautions were taken and tests given to assure the surgeon that you were in proper shape for the operation.

The laryngectomy was done, and you were amazed that you felt little or no pain during or following the procedure. You knew you were breathing more freely. You were fed liquids until the doctor knew your throat had healed enough for you to be given solid food. Your appetite was good. You tried to speak, but not a sound came out. You also found that you couldn't whistle and that your senses of smell and taste were less sharp. But you didn't let that discourage you. You had been told that as you recovered and learned to speak again, both these senses—not to mention the ability to whistle—would return.

At some time during your hospital stay, a stranger may have come to see you. He looked healthy, was very cheerful, and spoke to you easily in a low clear voice. He explained that he, too, had had a laryngectomy and that he had been asked by your surgeon to visit you. You were amazed at how well he spoke, sounding far better than you did before your surgery. You looked for scars or signs of the operation but saw none. There he stood smiling, talking, and full of assurance that you, too, would someday do the same.

He was wearing a collar and a tie which he now proceeded to undo to show you the stoma and how easy it was to conceal. He left, and his visit left you in high spirits. You had seen living proof that it was possible to assume your rightful place in life just at the point when you had thought you would have to leave off. That man was an image of the self you would soon be.

Now you have been discharged from the hospital and are back home again. Your doctor will have set a date for your follow-up examination. Don't forget it. It is of the utmost importance to go for regular checkups. Naturally if you feel any discomfort before the date of your appointment, get in touch with your doctor immediately.

You are feeling well; your appetite is good; and you're gaining weight. But at times you feel lonely and sorry for yourself. Some of these feelings stem from your inability to express yourself in words. It has made you withdraw somewhat, and you've been avoiding your friends. This is wrong. Now is the time to see your friends and to enjoy yourself as much as possible. Your friends are the same friends they have always been, and they're cheering for you. Don't be idle when you're alone, either. Read, get out and around; do some gardening if you like. Don't be afraid to exercise moderately. It'll be good for you. Most of all, don't indulge in morbid or gloomy thoughts.

You must remember that you have had a lifesaving operation. The troublesome growth has been removed, and you are in better health now than you have been for a long time. Perhaps you're asking yourself, "When am I going to talk?" This is different for each person. Let your doctor tell you when he feels you're ready. And then don't put it off. The sooner you start, the better. Remember, the more effort you put into it, the greater will be your reward.

As you proceed in your speech lessons, try not to get discouraged or worry about your progress. Don't compare yourself with others. Every person who has been laryngectomized is different, both physically in terms of the anatomy of the throat following surgery, and psychologically. Some grasp esophageal voice techniques quickly. Others take more time. Don't lose sight of the fact that you have a lifetime to live with your new voice and that the more time you now devote to developing it, the better it will be. You have a fight ahead of you to regain the power of speech. It will call for courage, persistence, and good humor all the way to a successful completion of the course.

Will I Go Back to Work?

THAT QUESTION has probably occurred to you many times since you became ill and had your operation. That, and perhaps "Will I be able to do the same work I did before?" The answer to both questions is usually yes. In a few instances your doctor may feel that your old job exposes you to some risk—dust or particles in the air, for example—which would be injurious to your health.

When that happens, there is always a state or federal agency that will be interested in your case and will either help you find other work or train you for another type of job. There is no reason why you can't work if you want to. This includes occupations that require a lot of talking: salesmen, teachers, supervisors, administrators.

Indeed, teachers of laryngectomees who are themselves

laryngectomized are prime examples of people who use their new voices a great deal. One of the pioneers in this respect was John Davis, a prosperous lawyer who was operated on in 1930. He taught himself to speak again and returned to the practice of law. He also began to teach other laryngectomees, and in the course of the next two decades taught over four hundred people how to speak. His pupils ranged in age from nineteen to seventy-eight, and he never had a pupil who failed to learn to speak. He did this on his own time and at his own expense. He also organized a Lost Chord League in Brooklyn.

Here are some other case histories:

A. M.—A U.S. army colonel, operated on several years before World War II. He had retired but was recalled to active duty and performed service of the highest value to the country.

T. C.—Continued in his position as a locomotive engineer on a large railroad.

A. L.—A high school French teacher, operated on in 1960. Six months after surgery, she was back in the classroom again.

J. B.—Taught himself to speak after surgery and continued to operate his stationery store in the busiest section of a large city.

R. C.—Editor of a business magazine. Relearned speech and resumed the hectic schedule of administration, writing, and editing.

C. W.—Went back to his position as a top-ranking insurance salesman.

W. D.—Continued for many years as a surgeon and director of a hospital.

J. L.—Sold his business because of chemicals and dust. Opened a stationery store which he ran successfully.

J. H.—Middle-management executive for a state telephone company. Constantly uses the phone or is in direct conversation with others.

J. K.—Dispatcher for a large trucking company.

M. M.—Still engaged as a salad chef in a large restaurant.

F. L.—A very busy building contractor who takes personal charge of all jobs.

S. M.—Continues to be one of the best dramatic coaches in the country.

H. M.—Owns and operates a horse ranch. Personally breaks in his horses.

V. P.—A busy general practitioner and surgeon who makes it a point to do a little extra checking if a patient complains of a sore throat.

D. L.—A secretary to a busy executive, she also administers a large typing pool.

L. S.—Saleswoman at an exclusive New York department store.

D. T.—A state trooper now working at a desk job.

And so on. The examples could be multiplied a thousandfold. Some of these men and women are in high positions; others are in more modest ones. All had the same desire to forge ahead. All refused to accept defeat or assume a lesser place in life. If you have confidence in yourself and the will to put up a fight for what you want, the chances are excellent you'll succeed.

How You Speak

THE LARYNX IS SITUATED at the upper end of the windpipe, or trachea, the hollow tube that leads down into the lungs. The larynx contains two elasticlike tissue folds, the vocal cords. Before your operation, when you breathed in, the lips of the cords were wide apart. This allowed air to flow in freely to fill your lungs. When you wanted to speak, the lips of the cords contracted. This brought them close together, so that the air, coming up from your lungs, had to force its way across your vocal cords. This force of air set the cords vibrating. It is these rapid vibrations that are the source of sound. As the vibrations spread out, striking the many resonating areas of your head and body, they were modified into tones and turned into speech sounds by the movements of your mouth, lips, and tongue.

Now your vocal cords have been removed, and the air that used to pass across them has been diverted. Both the incoming air you need to supply your lungs with the oxygen vital to life and the outgoing air pass through the opening in your neck—the stoma. This air is of no immediate value to you in the production of speech. You must, therefore, find some other source of air power and some other tissue to set into vibration in order to produce speech.

In most cases the surgeon has only removed the larynx and diverted the trachea to its new opening in the neck. He has left all the other mechanisms for making speech along with some scar tissue. What you have to do is to get some air into the back of your mouth and down into the upper part of your esophagus. This is your food pipe—that other hollow tube that lies behind the trachea and leads from the throat to the stomach. Trap air in the esophagus, and you have your new air-power source. Then bring that air up to vibrate against the tissue folds, muscles, and scar tissue at the junction of the esophagus and throat, and you have your vibratory center for producing sound. You can turn this sound into speech in the same way you used to before the operation.

Even now you are able to draw in and expel tobacco smoke, blow out a match, and make sibilant sounds like "sleep" or "shush" just by compressing air through your lips. To do this, some air must be entering your nose and mouth to supply the necessary pressure. You can draw on this same air to fill your esophagus. The various ways to do this will be spelled out in a later chapter. They are all means to the same end—to speak again by means of esophageal voice. As you practice, you will find that you will be using muscles you never used before. You'll become conscious of how your stomach, diaphragm, and chest muscles can be called into play, to help trap air in the esophagus and bring it up again to vibrate against the tissues of your new vibratory center, so that it can be formed into speech.

In the beginning you'll concentrate on air intake, learning how to fill the esophagus efficiently and quickly so you can do it whenever you want. At the same time you'll practice bringing that air back up again quickly to make simple vowel sounds like "ah" and "oh." Gradually you'll be able to extend your vocal powers so that you can say two- and three-syllable words on one air "charge" or breath, and eventually, whole sentences of eight to ten syllables.

As you master the technique, you will gain control over every step in the process. One, you will be able, consistently, to get air in quickly. Two, you will be able to bring it up rapidly to start vibrating. Finally, you will articulate clearly and smoothly so that you can say a whole phrase or sentence on one breath. The result will be a smooth, natural-sounding voice. You'll find yourself speaking in a style and rhythm that is part and parcel of your personality.

The Artificial Larynx

AT SOME TIME during the course of your illness, you have probably heard that there are special mechanical or electronic devices which can make speech possible for a laryngectomized person. Such aids are called artificial larynges. You may decide you want to try one, especially in the first days and weeks after surgery when you desperately want to communicate but are not ready to begin esophageal speech lessons. There's no reason why you shouldn't.

A while back, that last sentence would not have been written. It was thought that using artificial means would make it difficult to learn esophageal speech. The idea was that you would become accustomed to using this "crutch" and never be able to speak under your own power. This is not true. There are some people who may *prefer* to use a device, but anyone who sincerely wants to speak with esophageal voice will not be delayed in progress or hampered in any way by using such an aid.

Don't be put off by old-timers who frown on their use. The use of an artificial larynx will in no way deter you from learning how to speak, and it may be a great boon to your spirits not to have to rely on pad and paper, magic slates, gestures, or—worse yet—whispering. (Whispering is definitely out for the esophageal-speech student. It tightens up the muscles you're trying to learn how to control and makes it that much harder for you.)

The Pneumatic Larynx

A pneumatic larynx works something like a wind instrument with a reed. When you blow into a clarinet, the air pressure sets the reed vibrating, and by controlling your lips, the keys, and the holes out comes sweet music. One particular device has a reed or a flexible rubber diaphragm built into a small metal cylinder. Attached to the lower end of the cylinder is a tube that fits over the stoma. At the upper end is a flexible tube that you insert in your mouth. Air from the stoma supplies the power source that sets the reed vibrating. The vibrations are altered in the mouth to produce speech sounds. If you don't want to talk, you expose a small opening at the top of the cylinder. This allows the air to flow in and out of the stoma without vibrating the reed.

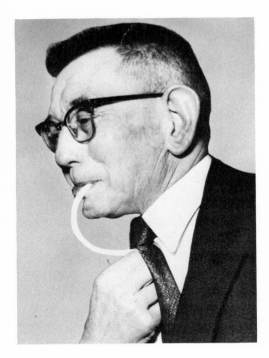

THE MECHANICAL
LARYNX

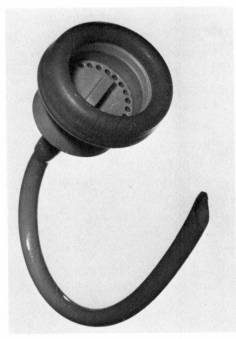

The Electrical (or Electronic) Larynx

Here the vibrator is packed into the head of a small
battery-powered instrument. The power unit may fit into a
shirt or jacket pocket, or the whole system may be built into
a cylinder as big as a medium-sized flashlight. When you
turn the switch on, the vibrator starts to buzz. It is placed
against the area of neck that is best suited to transmit the
vibrations across the tissue and into the mouth. This varies
from person to person, and you must find the area best for
you by trial and error. Again, the vibrations are modified by
the tongue and mouth parts to form speech.

There are a number of variations on mechanical and
electrical larynges available. One device manufactured in
England is actually implanted in a tooth. (Dental surgery is
necessary to make the installation.) Another is designed to
look like a pipe. There is a considerable range in price; the
most expensive are usually those that offer some ability to
change pitch (the highness or lowness of sound) to give
more variety to the voice.

One of the least costly battery-powered models is manufactured by Western Electric and available through the
business office of your local telephone company. It is a
hand-held cylinder with an offset head. This allows you to
position the vibrator optimally while holding your arm in a
relatively relaxed position close to your body.

It takes a while to get these devices. They all add their
own vibratory buzz or hum as background noise to your
speech. This is not too bad as you learn to control the
instrument, and it is less annoying when you speak on the
telephone. The microphone in the telephone will be more

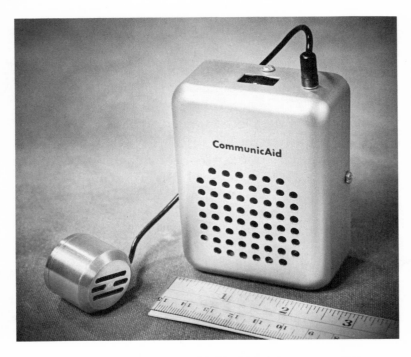

**POCKET-SIZE
ELECTRICAL LARYNX**
(Courtesy A. R. Mann)

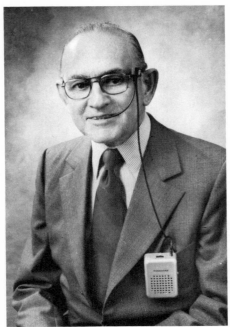

sensitive to the speech sounds coming from your mouth than the vibrations generated at the neck surface. Also the telephone filters out a lot of sound frequencies. (It is not a high-fidelity instrument.)

The artificial larynx, has a more limited frequency range than esophageal speech. It usually has to be hand-held, thus tying up the use of one hand. And, being a manufactured appliance, it can break down. The batteries have to be replaced. The device needs to be cleaned. Nevertheless, it does have a legitimate place in the life of a laryngectomee. It can be a godsend in the first few weeks when you're voiceless, especially if you're back on the job. It can also be a help when your own voice is weak because of a cold or fatigue. (There are also a line of voice amplifiers made especially for laryngectomees. They are very useful for the individual who can speak with esophageal voice but who works in a noisy surrounding or needs to be heard over a distance.) For those people who for one reason or another have difficulty in mastering esophageal voice, the artificial larynx is an invaluable substitute.

If you do decide to use one, you will need training. Many of the speech clinics or rehabilitation centers that teach esophageal speech also hold classes to demonstrate the various kinds of artificial larynx and to explain how to use each instrument. You need practice to find the right placement for the vibrator, to learn how to minimize vibrator noise, and to gain skill in articulating and phrasing, so that you get the very best quality of speech obtainable.

Insight and Outlook

BEFORE YOU START on your voice lessons, there are some things it will be helpful for you to know. They are based on the personal experiences of the author and many of his students.

You will find that until you are again able to speak, there will be some people who will shout at you or else go to the other extreme and whisper, making exaggerated lip movements. Both approaches are based on the general public's confusion that anyone who can't speak must be a deaf-mute. They don't mean any harm, but it can be very annoying. If it happens, just explain that you can hear quite well. That generally puts an end to the problem.

Then there are people who get annoyed at you! Once, before I regained my speech, I had occasion to take a taxi. I wrote the address of where I wanted to go down on a pad and handed it to the driver. Evidently he couldn't read. He shouted, "I can't read this. Why don't you speak, you dummy?" I was infuriated. A policeman finally came to the rescue and directed the driver where to take me. Although up to this time I had not yet tried to speak, I found that during the course of the argument a few words came out distinctly. The cabbie had done me more good than I realized. I was determined that never again would anyone say to me what he had said. Within a short time I was talking.

More than one laryngectomee has remarked that a little anger or annoyance triggered their first words. A few months after his operation, one man found himself snarled in bumper-to-bumper traffic on a two-lane road. "Damn!" he exclaimed, much to the surprise—and then delight—of himself and his wife.

One of my pupils spoke to me in class one day. He said he was depressed because the men in his shop cheered and clapped their hands whenever they were able to understand a few words he said. He thought they were making fun of him. I knew that the men were very fond of him and had been quite worried when he was in the hospital. Fortunately I was able to convince him that his friends, a group he had worked with for many years, were genuinely happy to hear him speak again. He began to see things in a different light and stopped being depressed. It's very easy to slip into a depressed mood. Try to guard against it.

Another time a pupil came up to me after several weeks'

instruction and said, "Do you think I'll ever speak again?" In amazement I said, "What do you think you're doing now?" She looked surprised and said, "That's right, I did say it, didn't I?" She had said a complete sentence of seven words, but the realization that she was actually speaking hadn't dawned on her. It takes us all a little time to realize we are talking.

Sometimes you'll find some people will hurry you along when you first start speaking. They're impatient and try to anticipate your next words and then say them for you. Usually they aren't the least bit interested in what you have to say. Keep away from them until you're speaking well enough.

When you go into a store to buy something, get as close to the counter as possible. Don't try to shout what you want, but ask for it as naturally as possible. You'll be surprised how sharply trained the ears of salespeople are. Every day they come into contact with people who have all kinds of different voices and accents.

After you begin to talk, some people are apt to remark, "Your voice is husky. Do you have a cold?" This is really very gratifying because it means they have no idea you have had to learn to speak in an entirely new way. You sound very normal to them. On the other hand, they are apt to follow up with some cold remedy Uncle Joe or Aunt Liz has been using for years and insist on writing it down for you. Don't bother trying to explain what's wrong. You'll get too involved, and before you know it, the story of your operation will lead to the story of their and their relatives' operations, and by the end of the discussion you'll feel you've also undergone their grandfather's appendectomy. Don't forget to throw away the remedy, either.

Some laryngectomees develop certain fears after the operation. I myself was afraid to drive a car. This worried me because I used to drive many miles a day and had driven every make of automobile. I was also a commissioned officer in a National Guard unit attached to a truck company. A short time after the operation, we were ordered to convey a battalion of troops to a camp for target practice. I was assigned to command the movement. I decided that this was the time to overcome my fear, and I received permission from my commanding officer to drive the lead jeep myself with no riders. I led the convoy of sixteen trucks to the camp, a distance of fifty miles, in an hour and a half, and returned to my home station with a motorcycle escort in an hour and a quarter. That freed me from all fear of driving. This doesn't mean you should burn up the road or take unnecessary chances, but it does mean that you should try to overcome your fears.

There are many other kinds of fear some of us develop. With some it's traveling; with others it's going to a show or a restaurant. When asked why they were afraid, they all said it was because they might cough and someone would notice them. This is unrealistic. Why should you cough more doing these things than when you're sitting at home? It's because you think about it. If you did cough, 99 percent of the people wouldn't pay the slightest attention to you, and the other 1 percent would think you were blowing your nose.

Another fear I had after the operation was that I might choke on a piece of food or a bone. Knowing that it is almost

impossible to cough up anything through the throat, this fear is natural enough. The fear, however, quickly passes once you understand that even if something did stick in your throat you couldn't possibly choke to death: Remember you breathe through the stoma—the opening in your neck. Any obstruction in your throat can wait to be removed by a doctor.

Similarly some people worry when they go to bed at night that they may suffocate. They try to sleep on their backs or with the covers only partly drawn up. Again this is unnecessary. Your breathing is still under the control of a special part of your brain, just as it was when you breathed through your nose. This brain center is always in operation whether you're awake or asleep. It makes sure you get enough air, regulates the muscles in the chest and diaphragm you use in breathing, and sets in motion the automatic reflexes that wake you up or make you turn over or adjust the covers so that there is no interference with breathing.

In another part of this book I mentioned a train engineer. He told me that for quite a time after his surgery he was afraid to touch a locomotive. He would just stand around in the yard trying to get up courage to drive again. Finally the company put him on a light locomotive running around the yard. Within a week he was able to go back on his regular long run.

In addition to fears and self-consciousness, some people find themselves getting angry or resentful—the "Why me?" attitude. This is more likely to happen in the first few weeks after surgery when you're frustrated at being unable to speak and having to write everything down or rely on gestures. Instead of giving in to the anger or frustration, let it be a goad to get you going on speech lessons. Just as a traffic jam drove one man to utter his first word—a curse— you can harness that anger or annoyance into positive action. Once you start learning to speak, you'll find your anger or resentment will fade.

None of these things may ever happen to you. Everyone's experiences and internal feelings are different. But for those of you who at times do feel discouraged or angry, fearful or shy, I hope that the realization that others have had similar feelings and have overcome them will give you the courage and confidence to do the same.

Some Dos and Don'ts

COMMUNICATING WITH THOSE AROUND YOU, either with your own voice or with an artificial larynx, is a major step in getting to feel like yourself again—able to work, travel, play, and enjoy your family and friends. But there are a number of other things you can do, and some cares and cautions you should take, that will make life a lot easier and healthier for you.

Stoma care. While you were still in the hospital, your doctor or nurse explained the importance of keeping the stoma clean. Remember to use a handkerchief or a piece of cloth to absorb mucus. Don't use bits of paper tissue or

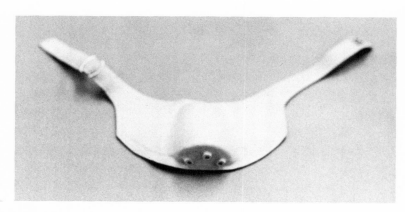

STOMA COVERINGS (Courtesy John McClear at I.C.D.) Top: A rubber stoma covering, for use in the shower. Center: An ascot and a turtleneck sweater front. These, or similar neck coverings, can be used by either men or women. Bottom: Women's jewelry that provides inconspicuous covering for the stoma. Necklaces of similar size and design can be easily purchased.

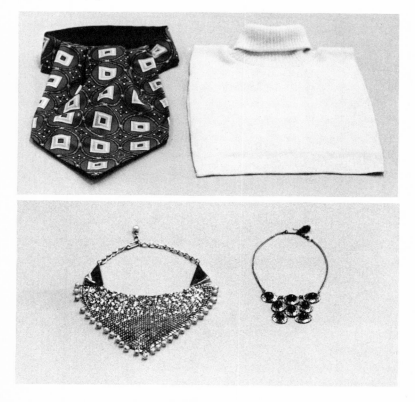

cotton balls. They are too lightweight or small and could be sucked up. If the surface is dry or crusted, use petroleum jelly, Albolene cream, or K-Y jelly to lubricate the edges. Always make sure your hands are clean first. Do not use olive, mineral, or any other kind of oil, baby lotions, or the like.

Wear a stoma bib or other light covering over the stoma. This is not just for appearance sake but as a health aid. When you breathed through your nose, the outside air was warmed, moistened, and filtered of dust as it passed through your nostrils and down to your lungs—a full two feet of airway. The stoma shortens that airway to about six inches, so there is far less opportunity for "conditioning" your air. A bib helps to do this. It creates an insulating space between the stoma and the atmosphere, so that the incoming air is warmed. The temperature differential also draws moisture from the air humidifying the stoma area. Finally the bib acts as a filter. Scarves, jewelry, turtleneck sweaters, and other wearing apparel can accomplish the same results. Keep the stoma covered when you go to bed as well. The same reasons pertain, but, in addition it is a courtesy to your bedmate. The bib will muffle any breathing sounds and also absorb mucus.

Collar Size. If a man normally wears a shirt and tie to work, he may find that after surgery the collar of his shirt is too large, that it has a disconcerting habit of slipping down and resting uncomfortably at the stoma level. To avoid this either move the collar button over, or if that isn't enough, see if you can't arrange to have your correct new size of collar sewn to the body of your regular-sized shirt. A custom shirtmaker will do this, and it is not terribly expensive. Check the yellow pages of your telephone directory to find who's available.

Bathing and Showering. These matters of personal hygiene are as important as ever, but in addition you can make use of them to relax and bask in a warm humid atmosphere that will do wonders for your stoma. The safest arrangement for the shower is to install a spray head below the level of the stoma opening. Or you might try one of the new hand-held spray attachments. If this is not possible, do not stand directly under the shower but some distance away and direct the spray as low as you can. You can also order a shower guard fitted to your neck size to protect the stoma from splashes (see Appendix I). Be sure to stand on a rubber mat, or have anti-skid strips fixed to the shower floor, and have grab handles conveniently placed.

If you prefer a tub bath, make it shallow. A half an hour in water hot enough to create a steamy atmosphere will do much to moisturize your airway. You can prevent the water from cooling off by setting the bath plug at an angle so that water flowing in equals the water draining out.

Shampooing and Shaving. These are not risky if sensible precautions are taken. The same kind of stoma shower guard can be worn when washing your hair in the bathroom sink or in the shower. Be chary with the shampoo and with shaving soap. You don't want a lot of rich runny lather that can run off toward the stoma. Men should shave carefully around the stoma, making sure to wipe away any loose hairs.

Weather Changes. Daily and seasonal changes affect the moisture and particle content of the air. If you find yourself coughing or producing a lot of mucus, it may be because of pollen or other particulate matter or because the air is dry. Coughing is a natural reflex that irritates the mucous membranes so that they produce more mucus. This helps filter out undesired particles and moisturizes the air. It's Nature's way of protecting your lungs. Use a humidifier if you live in a dry climate or if in winter your house furnace dries out the air. For temporary relief don't forget the virtues of a steaming tea kettle.

Sports and Hobbies. Water skiing, small boat handling, swimming, and other such water sports are out. There's just no point in exposing yourself to the risk. That doesn't rule out fishing from a large boat or from a pier or dock. Common sense also dictates against any body-contact sports. But that still leaves tennis, golf, bowling, skiing, and many other activities.

Follow-up Medical Appointments. Your doctor will remind you when he wants to see you. Make sure you keep these appointments. Naturally if you are having any difficulties, get in touch with him immediately. This is extremely important.

Personal Identification. It's an excellent precaution to carry with you at all times a Medic-Alert card or similar identification that indicates that you are a neck breather. Should you be in an accident and need artificial respiration, mouth-to-mouth resuscitation would be useless. The card will explain the first-aid measures to be taken to restore breathing to a laryngectomee.

EMERGENCY!

I am a Total Neck Breather
(Laryngectomee—No Vocal Cords)

I breathe ONLY through an opening in my neck, NOT through my nose or mouth.

If I have stopped breathing:

1. Expose my entire neck.

2. Give me **mouth to neck breathing only.**

3. Keep my head straight—chin up.

4. Keep neck opening clear with clean CLOTH (not tissue).

5. Use oxygen supply to neck opening. ONLY, when I start to breathe again.

BE PROMPT—SECONDS COUNT
I NEED AIR NOW!
(See other side)

Medical Problems
☐ Epilepsy   ☐ Glaucoma
☐ Diabetes   ☐ Peptic Ulcer
Other_____

Medicines Taken Regularly
☐ Anticoagulants ☐ Cortisone or ACTH
☐ Heart Drugs
   (Name and Dose)
Other_____

Dangerous Allergies
☐ Drugs (Name)
☐ Penicillin
Other_____

Other Information
☐ Hard of Hearing
☐ Speaks No English (Other)
☐ Wearing Contact Lenses
Other_____

NAME_____

ADDRESS_____

PLEASE NOTIFY:

NAME_____

PHONE_____

ADDRESS_____

CITY_____

OR

NAME_____

PHONE_____

ADDRESS_____

INTERNATIONAL ASSOCIATION
OF LARYNGECTOMEES

69-2R-50M-4/73-NO. 4520-PS   304

THE MEDIC-ALERT CARD. The International Association of Laryngectomees suggests you carry it at all times. In an emergency you might be unconscious or unable to give this essential information.

Moderation in All Things. That has been the advice of wise men throughout the ages and it applies in particular to the laryngectomized person. Don't overexert. Give yourself enough time to catch the train; don't race upstairs. Don't blow up when the waiter gets the order wrong or the soup is cold when you taste it. Once you're talking again, you'll find you'll be most comfortable speaking at a normal conversational level. Trying to raise your esophageal voice adds undo strain and makes it harder for others to understand you.

Moderation applies to eating and drinking as well. Follow your doctor's advice. If he says it's all right to have a cocktail or a beer occasionally, fine. But remember, alcohol tends to dry your throat and airway, and so can lead to discomfort.

Esophageal Speech—The Ways and Means

LET'S REVIEW what happens in normal speech. Air from the lungs flows up across the vocal cords. They are contracted and in close proximity, so they start to vibrate. These vibrations are the source of sound. (Remember, from your schooldays, that sound can't travel in a vacuum. You have to have a medium [like air], and the molecules of air have to be set into vibration to generate sound.) But if you can't control the vibration, the sound that emerges will be meaningless noise. So you use your throat muscles, your tongue, and your lips to shape your mouth and modify the vibrations so that what comes out are syllables, words, sentences.

A person without a larynx still has all the other parts

needed for speech, but must develop a new air supply and a new vibratory mechanism. The esophagus can serve as the new air depot. And the length of tissue connecting the throat (pharynx) and the esophagus, known as the pharyngeal-esophageal (P-E) segment, is your new vibrator. Once you've solved the problem of getting air down into the depot, and then back up vibrating over the P-E segment, you can produce speech in exactly the same way you did before. By shaping the parts of your mouth and moving your tongue and lips, you "articulate" to produce meaningful speech.

There is more than one way of getting air into the esophagus. That's very comforting because it means that there are a number of methods you can try to see which works best for you. Some teachers begin by just asking you to think about the problem: You have this great mass of air outside, and you want to grab a hunk of it and trap it into your esophagus. This may make you think of using your tongue as a shovel, letting it scoop up air and shovel it back into the esophagus. Others may think of this action as being like that of a piston and cylinder: the tongue is the piston bearing down on the cylinder of the esophagus.

A common association is that the action is like swallowing. It's not really swallowing because if you swallow air, it ends up in your stomach—and is no good to you as a source of speech, unless you can get it back up again into your throat. This is possible, of course, for that's what happens when you burp or belch: you bring up air from your stomach, and it makes a noise.

If you can mimic the action of swallowing air without

drawing it all the way down into the stomach, just get it into the esophagus and then return it in an esophageal burp, that does the trick. If in the course of postoperative recovery you found it easy to burp, or if as a child you could burp at will, you've got the problem licked.

Some students find they can get air into the esophagus by just opening their mouth and sucking air in. They don't have to move their tongues or go through a pseudo-swallowing motion. This is called the *inhalation* method, and it depends on controlling chest and stomach and diaphragm muscles. What's really happening is that you're creating a partial vacuum in the esophagus by pulling down on the muscles in your chest. In this way the outside air is pulled in to fill the partial vacuum.

Teachers use a variety of words to describe air intake. They may say you must get a "charge" of air, "pump" in air, "suck" it in, "inject" it, "gulp" it, "swallow" it, and so on. The words are loosely related to the various methods that work. X-ray motion-picture studies of esophageal speakers have greatly clarified the process, so that professional speech therapists can analyze the differences between one technique and another. Generally they classify the methods as

1. **Inhalation.** Air is sucked in through the mouth or nose. Tongue movements are unnecessary, and the esophagus is filled with air as a result of pressure differences created by chest and stomach muscles pulling down to create a partial vacuum in the esophagus.

2. **Injection.** Here various movements of the tongue are used to move the air back and down into the

esophagus. Since the Greek word for tongue is *glossa*, these methods are also called *glossal press* or *glosso-pharyngeal press* (depending on subtle differences in the tongue's action). Sometimes both the tip and the body of the tongue play an important part in the action. And in one method, not only is the tip of the tongue placed against the back of the upper teeth or gums, but certain consonantal sounds are also added, like *t* or *p* or *k*. These sounds are properly called "plosives": they are like little explosions in your mouth and can be made without vibration. They provide an extra force to help fill the esophagus. When they are used, the method is called *consonant injection*.

All these techniques for gaining air intake are efficient and you should use whichever one seems most natural to you. As you become more proficient in esophageal speech, you will find you use more than one method, depending on the circumstance. What's exciting is that they all become automatic and unconscious with practice. Eventually you will no more think about what you're doing than you did when you used your vocal cords to speak.

In the beginning, however, you will find you need to pay attention. You are trying to learn a new skill, and to do so, you must concentrate on what you're doing. You are learning to flex muscles you never used before and learning to control old ones—those in your chest, for example—in a new way. You may find it useful to use a mirror to watch what's happening as you practice. This will help you pin down what it is you're doing when you succeed in making a sound. When that happens, the first rule to follow is to try to do the same thing again—in that way you encourage the habit. Think of what you did, what you said to yourself, what your head movements were like. If what you did wasn't exactly a pumping action or a gulp or any of the other words your instructor used, use your own term for it. This is one part of speech training that is very personal and very hard to describe in words.

Try to relax all the time you're practicing. If you become tense, your muscles will fight you and make the battle that much harder. You needn't sit down. You may be more relaxed if you stand or move around. Try not to cross your arms or legs if you are seated as these restrict your body. It may help if you think of some natural action you do that involves pressing and releasing. A housewife found she was better able to produce sounds when she was doing her ironing at the same time—pressing down on the clothes.

As an added ploy, you can also sip soda or some other carbonated beverage, preferably warm, so that the bubbles are that much more active. Try the following:

Take a small amount of the beverage in your mouth and hold it.

Take a deep breath and hold it.

Swallow. (This locks the air.)

Now put pressure on the stomach and force the air back up through the P-E segment. The sound that comes up will be like a belch. Continue this until the sound comes easily, and you are able to get a sound each time. Form the sound into AHH. . . .

If you find that the soda causes too much gas, try plain

water. As soon as you feel you can swallow easily, do it without water. Now you're getting a feeling of the action and the sensation of a filled esophagus. The important thing is to get the air locked in the esophagus. Try to do this without completely swallowing it and having to bring it up from the stomach.

The Nelson Method

SEVERAL WAYS of getting air into your esophagus were described in the preceding chapter. Now I want to dwell on the method that I discovered worked for me and which I have taught many others. It does not involve swallowing air, so it is a comfortable technique that will not leave you feeling bloated. Naturally, if you experience difficulty with this method, try one of the others. The important thing is for you to develop speech regardless of the method you use. Don't waste time concentrating on any one technique if it doesn't seem to be going well.

My method is a variation of the glossal press. The air that enters the mouth and nose is locked in the throat by placing the tip of the tongue against the lower rear of the front gums of the mouth. The tongue is arched so that the center of the tongue touches the roof of the mouth just as if you were making the sound KUH. By pushing the arched part of the tongue hard against the roof and forward, a slight thump will be felt in the throat. When this occurs make a sound immediately before you lose the air that you have locked.

Practice with your tongue until you get the thump. There are other positions the tongue can be held in and still do it. Remember the position the tongue was in when you felt the thump and do it again and again. If the thump is very audible, put less pressure on the tongue muscles until you can lock the air without sound. Just lock it and say AHH. . . .

We do want to warn you, however, that when you are able to talk, you must say as many words as possible on one breath each time you lock the air, or else a sound will develop which will have come from taking in air in short gulps.

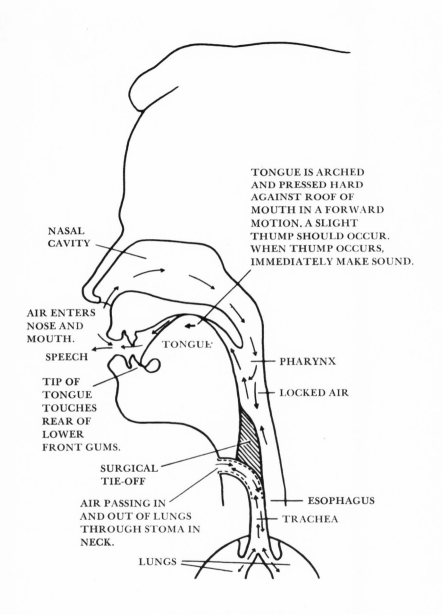

NASAL
CAVITY

TONGUE IS ARCHED
AND PRESSED HARD
AGAINST ROOF OF
MOUTH IN A FORWARD
MOTION. A SLIGHT
THUMP SHOULD OCCUR.
WHEN THUMP OCCURS,
IMMEDIATELY MAKE SOUND.

AIR ENTERS
NOSE AND
MOUTH.

SPEECH

TONGUE

PHARYNX

LOCKED AIR

TIP OF
TONGUE
TOUCHES
REAR OF
LOWER
FRONT GUMS.

SURGICAL
TIE-OFF

AIR PASSING IN
AND OUT OF LUNGS
THROUGH STOMA IN
NECK.

ESOPHAGUS

TRACHEA

LUNGS

THE NELSON METHOD

Lesson 1

AFTER YOUR OPERATION you may have been surprised at times to find you were able to say a good number of words quite distinctly. Those words were made up of sibilant sounds which you made by squeezing air through your mouth. Such words as sleep (you said *slp*), take (you said *tk*), sit (you said *st*), and many others are all said in the same way.

If you notice, all those sounds are consonants. When the surgeon removed your vocal cords, he removed your ability to make vowel sounds for which you need vibration: *a, e, i, o, u*, in their various forms, and also such semivibrating vowel sounds as *l, m, r,* and *ng*.

ā as in fāde	oi as in oil
ä as in ärm	ou as in out
a as in at	ū as in mūte
aw as in fall	u as in hut
ē as in wē	l as lll in Lil
e as in met	m as mmm in maim
ī as in mīne	n as nnn in nine
i as in fit	r (only one sound) as
ō as in hōme	rr in roar
ōō as in mōōn	ng as in sing

Practice these sounds. You have been told how they should sound. If in doubt, look back to see how they are indicated in the key words:

ā - ä - a - aw - ē - e - ī - i - ō - ōō - oi - ou - ū - u - l - m - n - r - ng

Before you start on another lesson, practice these sounds until you can say them easily. When you have mastered them, say the following: AWW. . . , UHH. . . , AHH. . . , IHH. . . , OOO. . . . Make these sounds as long and as loud as possible. This will strengthen your voice. Repeat them whenever your voice is weak. Repeat all the sounds in this lesson each day before you start on another lesson.

At this stage it's not advisable to try to make a long or complicated series of sounds. The important aim of the course is to get you speaking as quickly as possible by starting with the basic elements. We are not trying to correct your English, if it needs correcting, or to give you elocution lessons unrelated to your basic need to be able to speak again.

Lesson 2

YOU CAN NOW VIBRATE to produce tone. This tone can be turned into words by use of the mouth. Don't try to force the words out. Say them in a natural manner, after locking the air. Put a very slight pressure on your diaphragm.

at	not	no	cur	week
arm	met	pay	pack	care
me	able	pick	pad	cure
awl	ace	rope	bed	case
but	bear	rule	pill	use
oil	band	take	pew	tusk
cab	bar	too	pen	ton
cat	do	race	park	fun
fall	dab	roar	rob	trick

part	fan	red	rock	then
flew	fake	raft	tube	sick
sit	far	rare	tool	mine
out	get	look	trip	ten
note	jot	Lulu	type	maim
chin	Job	navy	saw	mail
boom	Luke	nine	way	mike
book	leap	nick	why	none
gun	mop	army	what	can

You are now on the brink of making speech. Sometimes you may think you'll never master it. Don't believe it. You have already demonstrated your talent by being able to say the words in this lesson. You have won the first part of the battle. In the same way you are going to go on with the lessons until the final victory of full speech.

At this point I must insist that you stop applying heavy pressure on your diaphragm. You want to gain control of your speaking air and develop a pleasing voice, not one that sounds like a belch. You may have noticed that the sounds and words you said in Lesson 1 were rather rough and that a blast of air could be heard coming out of the opening in your neck. At times, after locking the air, no sound came out at all.

The reason for the stoma blast was because you were trying too hard, putting too much pressure on the dia-phragm. When you couldn't make any sound at all, it was because in using that pressure you also pushed the locked air past your vibratory center, and it expended itself into nothing. It was wasted. If it did vibrate, it was a loud short blast of sound that was not understandable.

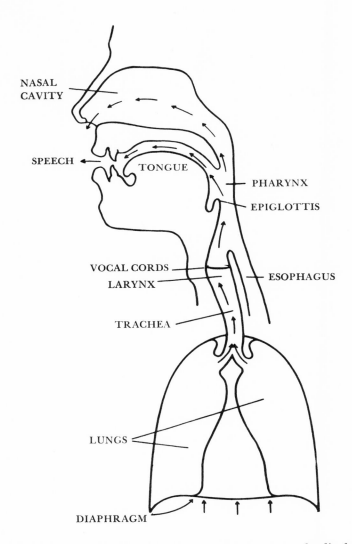

NASAL CAVITY

SPEECH

TONGUE

PHARYNX

EPIGLOTTIS

VOCAL CORDS

LARYNX

ESOPHAGUS

TRACHEA

LUNGS

DIAPHRAGM

BEFORE THE OPERATION when we put pressure on the diaphragm, we forced the air from the lungs up through the windpipe to vibrate against the vocal cords and come out of the mouth in the forms of speech. The greater the pressure on the diaphragm, the stronger the flow of air and the greater the vibration.

Applying pressure in this way is natural because it's what you used to do before your laryngectomy. The more diaphragm muscle power you applied, the more force was imparted to the air rushing over your vocal cords. The result was stronger vibrations which, in turn, meant louder sounds. (See the diagram on page 49.)

Control of Air

NOW IS THE TIME to begin controlling your speaking air. If you don't, your voice will continue to sound like a belch, and you will only be able to say a few words on each air intake. Once you start to control your speaking air, however, your voice will develop a more natural and understandable sound, and you'll be able to say more words on a breath. In the beginning, your voice may sound less loud to your ears, but it will be smoother and more distinct. Volume will come as you progress.

As a result of the operation, none of the air passing through your windpipe can enter your mouth. Instead it enters and exits through the stoma. If you apply greater pressure on your breathing muscles, you increase the noise of air escaping through the stoma. You get stoma blast, as it's called. But, as you know, stoma air cannot be used for speech. (See the diagram on page 53.)

To control your speaking air, do the following. Relax completely: "Stay loose," as the teen-agers say. Sigh very gently. If you still are getting stoma blast, you're sighing too strongly. Now sigh, and without locking the air, say AHH . . . to yourself. You don't hear any loud escape of air? Now sigh again, and on inhaling lock the air, and as you exhale it, say AHH. . . . Make the AHH . . . sound as long as possible until all the air has been gently expelled. You will notice that your voice has already lost the belchlike quality and taken on a more pleasant sound. Now go back and work on Lessons 1 and 2, and sigh out each sound and word in the foregoing manner. Always remember that whenever you hear stomal noise, it is caused by excessive pressure on the diaphragm. Stop completely and check to make sure you are fully relaxed. Then continue to sigh out each word. Do this from now on in all lessons and in all speech. In a short time it will become a habit as natural as walking.

Now try to lock the air with your tongue only *once* each time and speak, seeing how many words you can say on each air lock. When you've mastered esophageal speech you should be able to say five to ten syllables per each breath. When you are first able to do this, your voice may not be loud, but you will compensate for that by speaking smoothly and clearly. You will also lose the belchlike sounds. By practicing the exercises in Lessons 1 and 2, you will extend the range of your voice. By using the resonators described in a later part of the book, you will develop a richer and more natural quality.

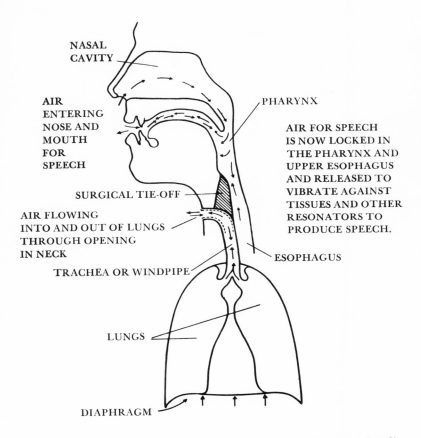

NASAL
CAVITY

AIR
ENTERING
NOSE AND
MOUTH
FOR
SPEECH

PHARYNX

AIR FOR SPEECH
IS NOW LOCKED IN
THE PHARYNX AND
UPPER ESOPHAGUS
AND RELEASED TO
VIBRATE AGAINST
TISSUES AND OTHER
RESONATORS TO
PRODUCE SPEECH.

SURGICAL TIE-OFF

AIR FLOWING
INTO AND OUT OF LUNGS
THROUGH OPENING
IN NECK

TRACHEA OR WINDPIPE

ESOPHAGUS

LUNGS

DIAPHRAGM

AFTER THE OPERATION, by putting heavy pressure on the diaphragm, you only drive the air out of the stoma in a loud noise and also
force out the locked air in the pharynx past the vibration points. In
doing this, you either produce no sound at all, or you produce a loud
indistinct sound. The surgical tie-off (shaded area) will not allow any
of the air from the lungs to pass through the mouth or nose. Neither
will the air entering the mouth and nose go to the lungs. Air from the
lungs cannot help you to speak. By putting very little pressure on the
diaphragm and breathing naturally and easily, you are able to control
the speaking air and avoid any unpleasant sound caused by escaping
air. In this way you give the tone of your speech a smoother and more
pleasant sound.

Lesson 3

COUNT IN THE FOLLOWING MANNER. Say each number on a single breath:

1 / 2 / 3 / 4 / 5 / 6 / 7 / 8 / 9 / 10 / 11 / 12 / 13 / 14 / 15 / 16 / 17 / 18 / 19 / 20 / 21 / 22 / 23 / 24 / 25

Now say the alphabet in the same way:

a / b / c / d / e / f / g / h / i / j / k / l / m / n / o / p / q / r / s / t / u / v / w / x / y / z

Did you realize when you counted that you were actually saying two- and three- syllable words when you reached the teens and twenties? Now say two numbers on a breath as given below. The space between the pairs denotes that a new breath is to be taken and locked before saying the next pair:

1,2 3,4 5,6 7,8 9,10

Now follow the same procedure with the alphabet:

a,b c,d e,f g,h i,j k,l m,n o,p q,r s,t u,v w,x y,z

Don't forget to go back each day and repeat the sounds described in Lesson 1.

On some days your voice may sound better than on others. Occasionally you may experience difficulty in locking the air or in bringing out words. This is typical of early learning. You will eventually develop consistency, that is, you will always be able to lock the air and bring it right back up again. At this time, however, you are consciously training your muscles. They may tighten up and resist you. Also you may be trying too hard, taking in too much air or not releasing it to best advantage. At the same time you may be exaggerating facial movements in an effort to speak clearly. The best thing to do is to stop what you're doing, relax, move around, or simply rest. The tendencies to strain, to lock in more air than you need, or to make facial grimaces are very common in the beginning. If you don't nip them in the bud, they can become bad habits.

When you feel refreshed, go back and repeat the sounds of Lesson 1.

Often you will find that shortly after a period of relapse,

your voice will sound better. Like the mouse climbing the well, you may always seem to slip back a halfstep before advancing a whole step. Don't let it worry you. Remember to stay loose. Even when you spoke with your normal larynx, if your stomach and chest muscles were tense, your voice sounded strained. Develop a habit of yawning occasionally. This relaxes your throat and facial muscles.

At this time the process of air intake is betwixt and between: It's not yet a fully automatic and unconscious habit, but you've made a lot of progress since the time you made your first sounds. If you concentrate too hard on the process now, you may find yourself in a situation comparable to watching your feet as you go down a flight of stairs: you may trip! What you want to do is to have your intake become as natural and smooth a body function as walking or eating. Sure, you must pay attention as you master it—but not too much!

Lesson 4

YOU SHOULD NOW be able to say two words on a breath. Be sure to say both words distinctly. Remember to sigh and not to push out the words. Check yourself for stoma noise. If there's too much diaphragm pressure, you won't be able to utter the second word clearly. Now say the following:

I am	it snows	two boys
sit up	right way	book end
flew in	feel it	new fad
get out	they are	black hair
you are	she is	row boat
had it	how far	say it

blue sky	red coat	how fast
it's his	man made	oil can
steep hill	nice boy	too sick
ink spot	sun shines	ten men
we are	run away	tom cat
he was	bull dog	run up
so near	big car	fat man
pick up	auto race	ask me
chin strap	in part	rare meat
use care	bank note	high bar
too much	new rope	heavy fog
it always	good job	you will
red hut	he said	fix it
gun shot	lost it	

Blend words when possible; for example, I (y)am, runaway.

Be sure that both words are said so that they can be easily understood. If possible, have someone listen to you and repeat what he or she hears.

Try to realize that you are now actually speaking.

Count in the following way. As before, each separation between groups means a new breath.

$$1,2,3, \quad 4,5,6, \quad 7,8,9, \quad 10,11,12,$$
$$13,14, \quad 15,16, \quad 17,18, \quad 19,20$$

Then the alphabet:

$$A,B,C, \quad D,E,F, \quad G,H,I, \quad J,K,L,$$
$$M,N,O, \quad P,Q,R, \quad S,T,U, \quad V,W,X, \quad Y,Z$$

Regaining Your Sense of Smell

AFTER THE OPERATION, you may have noticed that you have difficulty in recognizing odors, except a very strong one like gasoline. As you learn to speak and more air circulates in your nose and throat, it will help to stimulate sensation. You can further develop the sense by doing the following:

Take a bottle of perfume or a bar of scented soap and hold it to your nose and sniff it. You may or may not be able to smell it. Keep it in that position and lock the air as you do when you speak. Say a short AH—and immediately sniff the article again. To your surprise you will now be able to smell it.

Do this several times a day, using different articles each

time. Be careful not to use any strong chemical that might irritate the nasal passages. By doing this regularly, you will find your sense of smell greatly improved. As your speech improves and you carry on conversations more often, your sense of smell will become nearly normal. And since the sense of taste is partially influenced by smell, you'll find your taste buds reacting more normally as well.

One of my pupils had been a well-known prizefighter before the operation. For ten years prior to his surgery, he had been unable to smell as a result of a broken nose. I explained the above procedure to him, and much to his surprise he found that after all those years he was able to regain his sense of smell.

Lesson 5

ONLY IN PRINT is there a distinct separation of words. Spoken words come forth in a continuous stream, being pushed and pulled forth by the air. A break in a word or sentence only occurs when you shut off the air supply.

If when you drove a car, you put your foot on and off the accelerator in short bursts, the ride would be very bumpy and unpleasant. The same thing happens with your voice. If you fail to say as many words on a breath as possible and fail to keep just a slight pressure on the diaphragm, you will find your words bumping and jerking. By not breathing naturally, you develop an unpleasant sound caused by the gulping of air.

When you are asked to breathe and speak naturally, it means that you should try to breathe and speak exactly as you did before the operation. The only difference now is that you must first lock the air.

Take the number 75, for instance. If you drag it out as "seven-tee fi-ve," it will end up sounding like "seven-tee fi." The last part, the "five," will fade away; because you ran out of air before the entire number was said, a listener will be unable to understand what you have said. Yet before the operation you said "seventy-five" with no break between. Why shouldn't you do the same now?

Practice saying the following numbers exactly as they are written:

eleven	oneeleven
twentytwo	onetwenty
thirtythree	onethirty
fortyfour	oneforty
fiftyfive	onefifty
sixtysix	onesixty
seventyseven	oneseventy
eighteight	oneeighty
ninetynine	oneninety
onehundred	onethousand
onetwentysix	twothousand
sevenseventyseven	threethousandsix
fivefiftyfive	fourthousand
eighteightyfour	fivethousandfive
ninesixtyone	eightthousandone
twotwentytwo	seventhousandseven

threethirtythree   onehundredthousand
oneOone   threehundredfortyseven

Say the following short sentences as they are written.
(Those on the left are in the form in which they should be
read; those on the right are in the form in which you should
say them.)

READ	SAY
It ran away.	itranaway.
I saw it go.	Isawitgo.
We went out.	Wewentout.
So be it.	Sobeit.
Not for long.	Notforlong.
How are you?	Howareyou?
We ate rice.	Weaterice.
I believe it.	Ibelieveit.
There's none.	There'snone.
It is black.	It'sblack.
Where are you?	Whereareyou?
She is in.	She'sin.
The car runs.	Thecarruns.
I feel fine.	Ifeelfine.
He is good.	He'sgood.
We are home.	We'rehome.
Far far away.	Farfaraway.
Bring it along.	Bringitalong.
Hang it up.	Hangitup.
Sing a song.	Singasong.
It's raining hard.	It'sraininghard.
I can talk.	Icantalk.

| So high up. | Sohighup. |
| The light is out. | Thelight'sout. |

Did you notice how different and more understandable your speech was when you said the words without hesitation on a single air intake? Do this whenever you speak. The more words you can say distinctly on one breath, the better your voice will sound. Your ears are accustomed to the pace and style in which you spoke for many years before your operation. Don't change your method of speaking now. As was noted earlier, these lessons are not intended to correct your grammar or change your accent. They are designed to restore to you your natural way of speaking as soon as possible.

You can do only one thing at a time. If you want to change your accent or feel that your pace was too slow or too fast in the past, or if you use a lot of slang or improper English, don't try to correct it now. You can work on it at a later date, after you are able to speak with ease, by studying with a speech expert or English teacher or through self-correction. Just be natural now and do nothing that will interfere with your progress.

Lesson 6

AN IMPORTANT THING to watch out for after you are able to speak again is a tendency to become careless in articulation. Words or sounds that you form with your mouth and compressed air may get slurred because you have been concentrating all your effort on vibratory sounds. If you become careless in articulating, people will have difficulty understanding you. If, for example, you fail to make the compression shape of TH when you say THEY, it will come out EY; SHE will sound like EE; EXACT will become EYAC; and PUT will be a meaningless UT. Articulation means uttering distinct sounds by correctly using the tongue in relation to the other parts of the mouth and lips.

I will not spell out the precise position of the tongue in making most of these compression sounds, except in the case of S, SH, Z, and ZH. These are made by placing the tip of the tongue against the rear of the lower teeth and using the air that is within the mouth to make the compression sounds of S and SH, and the vibrating compression sounds of Z and ZH.

Some people disagree with me and feel the tongue should be in an upper position, but my experience is that these sounds are the hardest for you to make, and because of your low compression, they can be made much better with the lower part of the mouth. If, however, you feel you can make them better with the upper part, do so. After all, you said these sounds for many years before the operation, so just say them now in the same way, but be sure that each word or sound receives its full value and is said distinctly.

pop	Bab	fifth	vivid	wise
paper	baba	fife	viva	wire
poppy	baby	fifteen	vivify	write
papa	babble	fiction	vision	wren
pup	baboo	file	vizor	was
papal	Bub	fell	vocal	wring

white	they	tot	Dad	church
while	them	test	deduct	choice
whole	theme	tetra	deduce	chance
whim	thesis	Teuton	deed	chain
whiff	thanks	text	dude	cherry
whey	though	textile	dud	chess

joy	like	Nancy	yam	kennel
Jack	lilac	nanny	yard	kick
jade	Lily	nine	Yankee	kidney
jar	lilt	ninny	yokel	kirk
jail	limb	nip	year	kite
jest	limp	noon	youth	khaki

queen	sing	gag	king
quick	fling	gargle	ming
quince	having	gauge	fighting
quinine	leaving	gave	saving
quilt	wanting	gain	loving
quaint	going	glove	bringing

Be sure not to cut short the words ending in *ing*. If you do, the ending, *ing*, will sound like the word *ink*.

X ray	zoo	shush	suspends	budge
exact	zero	shawl	ceases	judge
flex	pause	slush	seizes	lodge
expend	cause	splash	suspects	dodge
packs	zebra	shave	sustains	fudge
facts	azure	plush	systems	badge

From now on, be sure that every word gets its full value. Don't start the next lesson, which consists of short sentences, unless you are certain you are now able to say every word distinctly.

Say the alphabet in the following way. (Remember that each space between a group of letters represents a breath.)

a,b,c,d,   e,f,g,h,   i,j,k,l,   m,n,o,p,   q,r,s,t,   u,v,w,x,
y,z

Count:

1,2,3,4,   5,6,7,8,   9,10,11,12,   13,14,15,
16,17,18,   19,20,21,   22,23,   24,25

Don't forget to go back to Lesson 1 for tone.

The Resonators

THERE ARE MANY RESONATORS in the head that can be brought into play to give your voice a better tone and richer quality. To do this you have to project your voice so that it vibrates not only in the throat as it does now, but also up against the palate, the roof of your mouth, the frontal sinuses and skull. The chart on page 73 shows that you are now vibrating at points **a** and **b**. By following the method given below, the vibrations can spread out to the areas around **c, d, e,** and **f**.

To bring your voice up out of your throat and give it a better tone, you should first get it to vibrate against the uvula (point **c** on the chart). If you open your mouth and look in the mirror, you will see a conical piece of flesh attached to the soft palate or soft part of the roof of your mouth, and extending down at the rear of the tongue. This is the uvula. To get your voice to vibrate against it, do the following:

Gargle exactly as you were able to do before your operation, but instead of using liquid, use air. Lock the air as in speech and open the mouth and gargle out the sound AH. . . . Let it come out very slowly in a continuous AHH . . . until all air is exhausted. You will feel the uvula quiver and vibrate. Then do the vowels *a, e, i, o, u* in the same way, and then the short words in Lesson 2. You will immediately notice the change in the quality of your speech.

The next step after you have mastered this is to bring the head resonators into play (points **d, e,** and **f** on the chart). You do this in a way similar to the way you were able to talk through your nose before the operation. To understand this, hold your nose and say HUMM . . . making it a long continuous sound. When this has been properly done, you will feel pressure inside your nose, and the sound will be very low.

Now release your nose and direct the sound in the same manner, still using the sound HUMM. . . . Place your fingers lightly between the lower bony structure of your nose and cheeks, and you will feel the vibration, if the sound is being properly directed. Practice this until you have no trouble in directing the sound and always keep it in the same areas. You will notice the improved tone of your voice and how nearly natural it sounds. Whenever you feel that your voice has slipped too far back into your throat again, repeat these exercises. In a short time, this will be a natural speaking procedure.

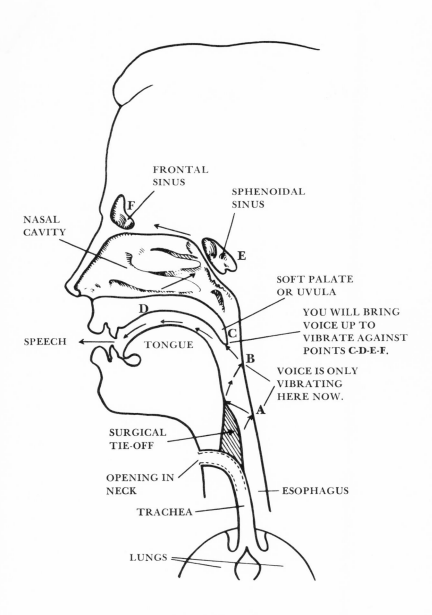

FRONTAL
SINUS

SPHENOIDAL
SINUS

F

NASAL
CAVITY

E

SOFT PALATE
OR UVULA

D

YOU WILL BRING
VOICE UP TO
VIBRATE AGAINST
POINTS **C-D-E-F.**

C

SPEECH

TONGUE

B

VOICE IS ONLY
VIBRATING
HERE NOW.

A

SURGICAL
TIE-OFF

OPENING IN
NECK

ESOPHAGUS

TRACHEA

LUNGS

THE RESONATORS

Lesson 7

EACH OF THE PHRASES given below contains four words. Don't try to push the last word out. Lock the air and speak naturally. Check yourself for any unwanted air sounds escaping through the stoma. If you have difficulty with any one sentence, skip it and go on to the next. Later, go back to the one you had trouble with, and you'll find it will be easier to say. Like many other things you've studied, if you work too long on one part without success, you're likely to get tired or irritated.

Repeat the following:

A word to you.
So many dream of.

I'll tell you all.
A real good time.

She's going to.
They have sent her.
As good as mine?
I'd seen it there.
Why are you here?
That's all for now.
They don't have it.
You think you are.
Isn't there a song?
I may see him.
Don't look up now.
We sit and talk.
It's too late now.
How'd you get it?
We've got plans.
I took a chance.
Let go of me.
This is so easy.
Stop there and ask.
Let's ask someone.
How're you now?
Do you want me?

My car is ready.
Only five miles away.
The driving is bad.
Twenty-four hours ago.
She was right there.
Come up here, please.
How'd you get it?
You stay at home.
I think there is.
Out of her heart.
He wants to go.
Where are you looking?
I'll just go home.
A very nice way.
It's why you called.
You pushed the chair.
Have you a match?
I think we're lost.
This must be it.
Want to save time?
Did you go out?
Where did you go?

When you ask a question, try to put the same expression into your voice that you did before the operation. That means letting your voice rise at the end of the sentence. But if you have difficulty getting that rising inflection, don't let it get a rise out of you!

Lesson 8

SAY THE FOLLOWING sentences. (The diagonal line between each group shows where a breath is to be taken.)

Through the long / night the / lathes turned.
Those things have / the exact size.
At the booth / was served / frothy broth.
Blow the bubble / out of the / bubble pipe.
For many months / the lilac bush / has
   been down.
People of many / faiths have found / a
   welcome.
The chess players / had their choice / of
   tables.

In the hall / his many dogs / were barking.
The Queen was / clothed in / expensive
  silks.
Many dads left / their hearths / to serve
  him.
Many deaths were / reported because of /
  no quinine.
Nancy and / the judge / went to church.
The clothes were / made of / excellent
  textiles.
A shell fell / between them which / was a
  dud.
The quince jam / was put up / in quaint jars.
Breathes there a man / with soul / so dead.
The prisoner served / many years on / a
  chain gang.
He was happy / singing / laughing / and
  playing.
Ill gotten money / is soon gone.
A long path / was cut through / with a
  scythe.
The flowers / in the park / had vivid / colors
  of red.

When you have finished this lesson, you should, during a
conversation, be able to say a larger number of words on a
breath. Speaking is usually easier than reading. At times
you will find that you can say from five to seven words on a
breath. Be careful that you don't go past your limitations.
See that each word remains understandable. It's better to
say one word less than to have the last word fade into

nothing. This matter is more fully described in Lesson 9.
Say the following numbers as written:

1,2,3,4,5,   6,7,8,9,10,   11,12,13,14,
15,16,17,18   19,20,21,   22,23,24,   25,26,27

Then say the alphabet:

a b c d e f g h i j k l m n o p q r s t
u v w x y z

The Telephone

YOU SHOULD now be able to talk on the telephone. No doubt you will be hesitant the first time. Rest assured that if you try, your voice will be quite clear and distinct. It's important for you to do this because it will increase your self-confidence. You'll realize you really are speaking and being understood.

The first time you use the phone let a friend or relative know ahead of time that you're going to call. That way they'll be expecting you and won't rush you. Take your time when you speak and hold the instrument just as you did before the operation. Don't try to talk too loud or force the words out. Speak naturally. The telephone will actually amplify your words. If for some reason you need the help of the operator in placing the call have someone else do it for you. Don't lock air to prepare for speaking until the person at the other end of the line answers. Then say what you want.

Lesson 9

As LONG as the number of words you can say on one breath is limited to three or four, you must be sure to group them in a way that makes sense to the listener. If you were to say: "We are going to a chop / house for a big steak," you would only confuse your hearer.

The point is that you must not try to say more words on a breath than you're up to. You could probably say "We are going to" quite distinctly, but "a chop" faded into no sound because you didn't take a new breath. You cut "chophouse" in half, so that with the next breath "house for a" came out clearly, but "big steak" was again lost.

You could have made the sentence sound sensible by not overreaching yourself and pausing as follows:

We are going / to a chophouse / for a / big steak.

If you don't go beyond your limitations and do not decapitate your words, you will be far more easily understood. As your duration time improves (the length of time you can speak on one breath) you'll find you'll be able to say:

We are going to a chophouse / for a big steak.

That's eight syllables on the first breath.

Later on, you'll be able to say the entire sentence on one breath. Meanwhile, you must plan out what you're going to say so that you can group your words into meaningful phrases. That way your listener will have no problem remembering what you have already said and will have a clear picture in mind. It won't be necessary to ask you to repeat.

The poem that concludes this lesson is an exercise in phrasing. Say it as it is written, remembering to take a breath where the slashes indicate.

THE CHILDREN'S HOUR

Between the dark / and the daylight, /
   When the night / is beginning / to lower, /
Comes a pause / in the day's / occupations, /
   That is known / as the / Children's Hour. /

I hear / in the chamber / above me /
  The patter / of little feet, /
The sound / of a door / that is opened, /
  And voices / soft and sweet. /

From my study / I see / in the lamplight, /
  Descending / the broad / hall stair, /
Grave Alice, / and laughing Allegra, /
  And Edith / with golden hair. /

A whisper / and then / a silence:
  Yet / I know by / their merry eyes /
They are plotting / and planning together /
  To take me / by surprise. /

A sudden rush / from the stairway, /
  A sudden raid / from the hall! /
By three doors / left unguarded /
  They enter / my castle wall! /

They climb up / into my turret /
  O'er the arms / and back / of my chair; /
If I try / to escape, / they surround me; /
  They seem to / be everywhere. /

They almost / devour me / with kisses, /
  Their arms / about me entwine, /
Till I think / of the Bishop / of Bingen /
  In his / Mouse-Tower / on the Rhine! /

Do you think / O blue-eyed / banditti, /
  Because you have / scaled the wall, /

Such / an old mustache / as I am /
   Is not a match / for you all! /

I have you fast / in my fortress, /
   And will not / let you depart, /
But put you down / into the dungeon /
   In the round-tower / of my heart. /

And there / will I keep you / forever, /
   Yes, / forever / and a day /
Till the walls / shall crumble / to ruin,
   And moulder / in dust away! /

HENRY WADSWORTH LONGFELLOW

Lesson 10

READ the following poem aloud. See that each line is said distinctly on a single breath.

THE FOUNTAIN

Into the sunshine,
   Full of light.
Leaping and flashing
   From morn till night.

Into the moonlight,
   Whiter than snow,

Waving so flower-like
  When the winds blow!

Into the starlight,
  Rushing in spray,
Happy at midnight,
  Happy by day!

Ever in Motion
  Blithesome / and cheery,
Still climbing / heavenward,
  Never aweary;—

Glad of all weathers,
  Still seeming best,
Upward or downward,
  Motion they rest;—

Glorious fountain!
  Let my heart be
Fresh, / changeful, / constant,
  Upward like thee.

JAMES RUSSELL LOWELL

Lesson 11

In this lesson the words of Lincoln's Gettysburg Address have been grouped to show you how many to say on each breath. Lock the air as quickly as possible, so the words will flow smoothly without too long a pause between them. Those pauses represent "latency"—the time it takes you to get air in and forced up again just prior to speaking. You want to work on reducing latency time.

Fourscore / and seven years ago / our fathers brought forth / upon this continent / a new nation, / conceived in liberty / and dedicated / to the proposition / that all men / are created equal. /

Now we are engaged / in a great / civil war, / testing
whether / that nation / or any nation / so conceived /
and so dedicated / can long endure. / We are met on / a
great battlefield / of that war. / We have come / to
dedicate a portion / of that field / as a final / resting
place of those / who here gave / their lives / that that
nation / might live. / It is altogether / fitting and proper
that / we should do this. / But, / in a larger sense / we
cannot dedicate— / we cannot consecrate — / we cannot hallow— / this ground. / The brave men, / living
and dead, / who struggled here, / have consecrated it, /
far above our / poor power to / add or detract. / The
world will / little note, / nor long remember, / what we
say here, / but it can never / forget what they / did
here. / It is for us / the living, rather, / to be dedicated /
here to the / unfinished work / which they who fought /
here have thus far / so nobly advanced. / It is rather /
for us to be / here dedicated to / the great task /
remaining before us— / that from these / honored
dead / we take increased / devotion to that cause / for
which they gave / the last full / measure of devotion— /
that we here / highly resolve / that these dead / shall not
have / died in vain— / that this nation, / under God, /
shall have a / new birth of freedom— / and that govern-
ment / of the people, / by the people, / for the people, /
shall not perish / from the earth. /

If you can say more words on a breath than we have
indicated for you, by all means do so. But don't sacrifice
clarity, and make sure your new groupings of words make
sense. Practice reading aloud from books or from the daily

newspaper. Do this at every opportunity that presents itself. If possible, have someone listen to you. Have the person sit behind you, so that there will be no way to read your lips. Repeat any word that sounds indistinct until you have pronounced it clearly.

You don't need any prescribed material to practice on at this point. That might only bore you. Instead choose material that interests you and read it aloud.

Do this often and get into discussions with friends or family regularly. If you are accustomed to speaking and reading a foreign language which is easier for you than English, do so.

Now You Can Speak

FROM HERE ON, you're on your own. This book has tried to show you how to speak again, and how you can improve the quality of your speech once you begin. More than that no book can do. You furnished the courage and the will power to win the fight and to you must go the credit for what you have accomplished.

Although you may now speak quite clearly, you must still practice to make your speech as near perfect as possible. Lessons cannot do this for you. You should use your voice at every opportunity and have confidence in your new power. Your speech will keep on improving each day you use it. At times you will find yourself trying to sing, and the result won't be bad at all.

Friends, relatives, and countless strangers you have encountered appreciate the fight you have made, and they have the highest admiration and respect for you. Something else has happened, too. You have acquired a warm glow of satisfaction within yourself, a glow that comes from the realization that you have overcome a handicap. You know now that there will never be any obstacle too big for you to overcome.

You find that you are more tolerant of people, and you have the urge to help others. You never look at handicapped people with anything but respect and admiration. You realize that they, too, have put up a fight to overcome great difficulties. You know that whatever handicap a person faces may also bring out the best that is in that person.

You never know who among your friends and neighbors may be the next to go through your experience. As it happened to you, illness may strike without warning. If it should, the person will suffer the same doubts and anxieties that you experienced. He or she will need someone like you to help when the going is rough. You can provide the same kind of assurance and lift to such a person as the author has tried, in this book, to give you.

You can do your part in helping others by working through a local Lost Chord club or by asking your surgeon if there is anyone about to undergo a laryngectomy who could benefit from a visit.

There are many things you yourself may discover that will hasten or improve your speech. Don't keep them a secret. Pass them along, so that others can profit from them.

After all, it was only by studying the actual experiences of laryngectomized people that the various methods for restoring speech were worked out.

You have a full life of good health and happiness ahead of you. Enjoy it!

Appendix 1

Sources of Information

YOUR GENERAL PRACTITIONER, surgeon, speech clinician, or a fellow laryngectomee who visited you during your hospital stay may have already acquainted you with local sources of information, instruction, or social contact with other laryngectomees. You may find that there is a Lost Chord club or similar organization nearby. Such a group can put you in touch with individual speech therapists or esophageal-speech training centers or may have members who are instructors.

If not, a good starting place for information is the nearest office of the American Cancer Society. The ACS has a variety of booklets, pamphlets and other materials. It is also affiliated with the International Association of Laryngec-tomees. This organization, founded in 1952, now repre-sents more than two hundred clubs for laryngectomized persons in the United States and abroad. Its directory is a source of information about products or equipment (such as artificial larynges), books, films, and other educational materials of interest to laryngectomees. In addition, it pro-vides a list of member clubs by city, giving the local ad-dresses of club officers. It can be obtained by writing to the IAL executive office in New York City: International Association of Laryngectomees, 777 Third Avenue, New York, New York 10017.

If there is a medical school or a good general library in your area, you may be able to borrow books or read articles on speech rehabilitation for laryngectomees. Some books written for public speakers or others who want to improve diction or articulation frequently contain useful word lists, tongue twisters, and other good vocal exercises when you feel up to it.

One such is by Grant Fairbanks: *Voice and Articulation Drillbook*, Harper & Row, New York, 1960. Another book with good exercises is *Self Help for the Laryngectomee*, by Edmund Lauder, available for $3.75 from Lauder, 11115 Whisper Hollow, San Antonio, Texas 78238.

John McClear's book, *Your Second Voice*, explains various methods of injection for the production of esophageal voice. In addition there are many anecdotes, hints, and advice about grooming, health, and so on. It is available for $5.00 from John E. McClear, 145 Center Avenue, Atlantic Highlands, New Jersey 07716.

For those interested in research and technical studies of

speech mechanisms in laryngectomized persons, there are professional texts. Among the best is by William J. Diedrich and Karl A. Youngstrom, *Alaryngeal Speech*, Charles C. Thomas, publisher, 301 Lawrence Avenue, Springfield, Illinois 62703.

Other titles are listed in the IAL directory and new titles continue to appear. Professional medical journals, such as the *Journal of Speech and Hearing Disorders, Laryngoscope*, and *Archives of Otolaryngology* carry current articles on esophageal speech or the rehabilitation of laryngectomized persons.

Appendix 2

Sources of Supplies

Stoma Coverings

A STOMA BIB or air filter is highly recommended not only for cosmetic reasons, but to filter, warm, and moisturize the air coming into the stoma. Local Lost Chord Clubs or the American Cancer Society can usually supply these, sized to fit your neck diameter. Instructions for crocheting bibs are available from the New York Anamilo Club, Speech and Hearing Institute, 340 East 24 Street, New York, New York 10010 and are also given in John McClear's book *Your Second Voice*. Instructions for making nylon bibs are available from the International Association of Laryngectomees, 777 Third Avenue, New York, New York 10017. Women interested in making scarves, dickies, and other neck apparel can write Teckla Tibbs, 1954 North Kenmore Avenue, #5, Los Angeles, California 90027 for how-to-do-it instructions. Other suppliers are listed in the IAL directory.

Shower Guards

A rubber shower collar is available from C. L. Sheldon, P. O. Box 128, Watertown, Massachusetts 02172. Plastic shields are available through the Lost Chord Club of Southern California, c/o Eugene Gerbereaux, 560 E. Villa Street (#824), Pasadena, California 91101.

Emergency ID

It's wise to carry on your person some form of identification indicating that you are a neck breather. The Medic-Alert Foundation, P.O. Box 1009, Turlock, California 95380, makes a bracelet. A pocket card is available through the IAL office. Your local American Cancer Society office also stocks these items (Code 4520). Auto stickers at $.15 each can be ordered from Arthur W. Collins, 7340 N. Hoyne Avenue, Chicago, Illinois 60645 (include cash with order).

Artificial Larynges

The following is a partial list of manufacturers of artificial larynges:

Luminaud Company, 7670 Acacia Avenue, Mentor, Ohio 44060

Makers of the Cooper-Rand Electronic Speech Aid. This consists of a pulse generator, containing circuitry and batteries, which fits into a shirt pocket. It is connected to a lightweight tone generator, which is held in the hand. A tube from the tone generator is inserted in the mouth when you wish to speak.

Western Electric Electronic Larynx Type 5

This is a small cylinder-shaped unit held against a suitable area of throat and activated by a battery on-off switch and an on-off and pitch-control knob. (This means that the battery can be switched on, but no vibratory tone is generated until the control knob is depressed.) The instrument is manufactured on a nonprofit basis and is available through the Bell System. (Contact the business office of the local Bell telephone company to order one.)

Cardwell Associates, Inc., P.O. Box 1135, Torrance, California 90505

Manufacturers of the *Verbalizer*, a battery-operated device, consisting of a power unit that can be fitted into the pocket and a cord leading to a small sound unit placed in the mouth.

Jedcom Products Ltd, 318 Green Lanes, London N4 1BX, England, distributed by Park Surgical Company, Brooklyn, New York

Makers of *Bart's Vibrator*, a self-contained battery-operated unit somewhat like the Western Electric model: It is a hand-held cylinder with an offset head containing the vibrator, which is positioned against the neck.

Dr. Kuhn & Co. GMBH, D 5000 Köln 91 (Merheim) Western Germany, distributed by Siemens Corporation, 685 Liberty Avenue, P.O. Box 1425, Union, New Jersey 07083

Makers of the electronic *Servox Speech Aid*. This is also a cylinder, tapered at the end, and held against the neck. The Servox offers some variation in pitch by varying pressure on a pitch-control regulator. It is said to provide more natural-sounding speech.

Voice Amplifiers

An amplifier may be helpful for a person with a weak esophageal voice, or for use when there is high background noise or if a cold or other illness affects esophageal voice.

The local Bell System business office can supply amplifiers. The Luminaud Company also makes an esophageal voice amplifier called the Rand Voice Amplifier.

Some other manufacturers are

CommunicAid Electronic Voice Amplifier, 1560 West William Street, Decatur, Illinois 62522

This unit packs a small microphone into a unit that can be fitted onto eyeglasses. Cords extend to the mouth and to the pocket battery supply.

Brenkert & Deming, P.O. Box 75, Royal Oak, Michigan 48068

Makers of Macrovox speaking aid and amplifier for weak voices. This consists of a tapered, cylinder-shaped, hand-held microphone attached to a power unit. (Like many amplifiers, it can be used by anyone with a weak voice, not only esophageal speakers.)